21 Simple Things You Can Do To Help Someone With Diabetes

Cherie Burbach

21 Simple Things You Can Do To Help Someone With Diabetes

All Rights Reserved

Copyright © 2009 by Cherie Burbach

Cover art by Cherie Burbach

Printed in the United States of America.

Also by Cherie Burbach

Nonfiction

Art and Faith: Mixed Media Art With a Faith-Filled Message

100 Simple Ways to Have More Friends

Glass Sculptures: How to Make Beautiful Sculptures for the Garden Using Vases, Bowls, and Other Glass Pieces

How to (Really) Make Money Blogging

Emotional Affairs: How to Prevent, Stop, and Move On From an Emotional Affair

Poetry

Poiema

Angel Toughness

My Soul Is From a Different Place

Father's Eyes

The Difference Now

A New Dish

New and Selected Poems

Yes, You

For more information please visit:
cherieburbach.com

21 Simple Things You Can Do To Help Someone With Diabetes

© 2009 Cherie Burbach

Table of Contents

Introduction

Why should non-diabetics get informed? Because as much as we know about diabetes treatment today, the support from our family and friends still plays a part in how healthy we are. An understanding approach from someone who cares means everything to us.

More than that, if you're around us enough there might be a moment when we could use your help. As someone who aims for tight control, I've had a time or two when my blood sugar has dropped low and a friend near me ensured I drank the proper kind of juice in order to get my blood sugar back to a healthy number.

The people in my life who really care about me understand things like an A1c test. They can genuinely sympathize when I tell them my blood sugar is running high or low. They know what the numbers on my monitor mean. A few, like my husband, can even give me shots and check my blood sugar. All of this helps me tremendously, and takes a mental burden off my plate.

And when you're diabetic, you often feel that help is at a minimum. You deal with insurance issues, misinformed people, and even medical personnel that seem apathetic at best.

So, thanks for taking the time to find out more about diabetes. In picking up this book, it means that you want to support your diabetic friend or family member. I've been diabetic myself now for twenty years, and have wanted to write this for a long time.

When I first became diabetic, I was amazed at how many times someone around me would hand me a sugar-free soda when my blood sugar was low, or investigate the food I had on my plate, or tell me I got the disease from eating too much sugar.

Everyone, it seemed, had an opinion or thought they wanted to share. The trouble was, very few people had good information about diabetes.

Diabetics deal with the fear of complications, burden of maintenance costs, and wear and tear on our bodies from organs that are overworked. Some of us deal with multiple needle injections. We deal with so much more than you would think.

Diabetes isn't just about "not eating sugar." Our blood sugars can change with stress and exercise and illness.

Your diabetic friend or relative counts on you to be the person in their life that "gets it" when no one else does. This book will tell you what you can do to help. Things like what you should (and shouldn't) say, what you should learn to truly be supportive, and even how you can help in the fight for a cure.

My hope with this book is to get you the information you need to be the very best friend to your diabetic pal.

This book is:
- a source of encouragement
- a prompt for education
- a starting guide to diabetic etiquette.

This book is *not*:
- a medical reference book
- a substitute for a nurse, doctor, or other medical professional.

In other words, this book *won't* give you medical information. It will, however, give you a starting point so you can find out what you should. The rest is up to you.

21 Simple Things You Can Do To Help Someone With Diabetes will point you in the right direction so you can truly support your diabetic friend.

#1
Learn About the
Disease

I mean, really find out all about it. You may think you know a lot about diabetes based on things you've heard or friends or relatives who have it. But unless you take the time to really understand the ins and outs of the disease, you won't know what you *should* know.

What I'm talking about here is getting some real education. Why? Because you can help your friend by being able to talk about diabetes in a way that is knowledgeable and helpful, rather than condescending, reproachful, or incorrect. While you wouldn't intentionally try to be judgmental or unhelpful, you probably would sound that way.

Besides that, there are so many new updates in the world of diabetes that you will be amazed at the medical information available.

It may seem daunting at first - what with all that talk about pancreatic function and insulin and injections - but when you understand what's happening in your friend's body, you will appreciate your own working pancreas all the more. When you gain the knowledge of what diabetes really is, you'll never again look at exercise, eating, stress, vision, and pain the same way again. More than that, you'll be better able to be truly supportive if you come from a place of knowledge.

#2
Know the Signs of Low Blood Sugar

This is one area where even the most independent of diabetics sometimes need help. When we are having an "insulin reaction" or low-blood sugar attack, we don't always think clearly. As the years have gone on for me, there are times when I am in the midst of an attack and for the life of me can't "get it" with my brain.

The reason it's important for *you* to know the signs is that you may need to help us. There will be times when our blood sugar dips so low that we can't reason through it and can't for the life of us remember what to do. Thinking becomes fuzzy. It doesn't happen all the time, but there are occasions when it will happen.

Understand the signs and be ready to act. Have sugar soda or regular juice ready to give us *regardless of what we say*. We may tell you we're okay when we're really not. Make sure we test our blood sugar before you leave us alone.

Ask your diabetic friend or relative where their testing supplies are. (They should always have them on their person.) Help them test (and learn in advance what the readings mean.) Then help them react.

Along with this advice comes the flipside: don't raid your diabetic's friend's juice or sugar soda stash! I used to keep juice in the bottom drawer of my desk and every day a guy I worked with would saunter over and say, "Wonder what's in your goody drawer today."

He acted as if the drawer in which I kept my sugar items was his for the taking. If he wanted a snack or some juice he'd help himself. Sure enough, one day I found myself having a low-blood sugar incident, and when I reached in my drawer to get my juice it wasn't there. The entire drawer was empty because he had helped himself one time too many.

As it was I had to run to the snack machine on the second floor and dig for change in order to get a sugar soda (which is really not the optimum method of raising your blood sugar anyways). I was covered in sweat and had to go home with the raging headache I got from allowing my blood sugar to slip so low.

The funny thing was, this guy *knew* I was diabetic. But he didn't get what it meant. After this incident I had to sit down with him and explain why it's so important that he not take the juice or candy out of my sugar drawer. He just shrugged because even then he didn't understand what the big deal was. He said, "You never even drink most of that juice. It just sits there."

Obviously he still didn't get it. But use his example of what *not* to do when it comes to your diabetic friend.

#3
Understand Diabetic Numbers

Sometimes diabetes can feel like a disease that's all about numbers: blood sugar, A1c, insulin dosage, carbohydrate grams....

One way you can help your diabetic friend is to understand what some of these numbers mean. For example, when your friend complains that his blood sugar is always 200 when he wakes up, understand that it means he or she is saying it's too high (and they probably feel lousy.)

If they are excited and tell you their A1c hit the magic 7 or below number, help them celebrate.

Understanding the numbers means you'll also be able to share the victories and disappointments with your friend.   You'll be better able to empathize and your friend will truly appreciate that you took the time to learn. It will make him or her feel as if there is one more person truly in their corner.

#4
Stop Judging

You'd be surprised at the things diabetics hear from people. Not only do we have to deal with the costs, stress, fear, and frustration in living with a chronic disease, we sometimes have to listen to people talk about how we "did this" to ourselves.

Here's the reality, I got diabetes when I was thin, young, and otherwise healthy. At the time of my diagnosis I worked out five times a week for two hours a day. I was just about to enter a run and bike race. I was in great shape.

Diabetes strikes all ages, genders, ethnic groups, and walks of life. It doesn't just strike people who are overweight or have not taken care of themselves. If that was the case every overweight person out there would have it.

The reason you shouldn't judge other people is simple: If you think you're "above" getting the disease, you're wrong.

More than that, however, if you really want to help your diabetic friend or family member, you can't look at them condescendingly. Your support is what matters to your friend, who every day deals with something you are lucky enough not to have. Your friendship and encouragement are what will help your friend succeed in managing his or her diabetes.

#5
Don't View Insulin as a Cure

Diabetes used to be a death sentence before the days of insulin. But just because insulin helps us to live from day to day doesn't mean it cures us from having diabetes.

I say this because I've dealt with many people that argue with me about research and funding based on their belief that diabetes already has a cure. It doesn't.

While insulin is a truly wonderful thing (and the reason I'm able to sit here and write this book), it doesn't mean that I'm cured. Oh, how I wish.

Not only is insulin NOT the cure but it's also some tricky business. Think about it, diabetics each and every day try and replicate what one organ does naturally in everybody else. And for those in tight control, a mere unit or two off and they can experience low blood sugars.

While we know so much more about types of insulin and dosage, the reality remains that we are still trying to work as our pancreas does, without the knowledge it has.

For example, if I eat an apple and sandwich, I have an idea of how much insulin I need for that based on my how many carbohydrates are in each item. But consider that I might be catching a cold that day, or I'm under extreme stress at work, or I haven't exercised as much as I usually do, or I've exercised slightly more than I normally do.... and my "guess" on how much insulin to take will result in a slightly higher or lower blood sugar number.

A normal working pancreas will know exactly how much insulin to kick out. It doesn't matter if the person is sick or has exercised or is under stress. In a healthy person, the amount of insulin is always perfect because the pancreas does the calculation for you.

In a diabetic, insulin dosage is based on knowledge of carbohydrates and a best guess. We can copy what our pancreas does, but we aren't going to be perfect. We need to do this calculation several times a day.

The other thing you need to realize is that insulin prolongs our life, and while we aim for tight control there are still no rock solid guarantees against complications. Tight control makes them far less of a reality, to be sure. But even with insulin, we still may have to deal with all those spooky complications. The longer we have the disease, the more real that danger can become.

Insulin is wonderful. It allows us to live. But it's not a cure.

#6
Retire From the
Diabetic Police Force

Just about every person with diabetes can share a story about someone who constantly monitors the food on their plate. They'll look at our carbs, amount of fruit, desserts, and comment on the items they see.

The problem? These people are usually way off base with what they think they know.

For example, I used to work with one woman who screamed at the top of her lungs each time she saw me eat more than one piece of fruit a day. If I had a banana for breakfast, and then a sandwich with apple at lunch, she'd say, "I'm going to tell. Diabetics can't have that much fruit. I know because my niece is diabetic."

If she would have listened to the first point of this book (learn about the disease), she would have known that diabetics most certainly can and should have fruit. Even more than one piece a day.

In the same office, I worked with an exceedingly thin woman who refused to eat a balanced meal but would instead drink four beers each night after work. She was obsessed with food (mine and anyone else's) and would comment on each thing I had on my plate. During a holiday party, I placed a small piece of cake on my plate and she came up to me and said, "Way to manage your diabetes!"

I told her my A1c was under 7 and I was doing just fine, thanks. She gave me a blank stare in return. Of course she didn't know what an A1c was! But she felt confident in commenting on my plate nonetheless.

I'm sure there are diabetics out there who don't pay attention to their diets. But the fact is, most of us do. We watch our blood sugars, we exercise, we try our hardest to maintain good control. So even when you think we are "cheating," chances are we simply living as normal a life as possible.

More than that, however, unless you truly know and understand the disease, your "policing" of other people's plates not only lacks intelligence but it's also downright rude.

Look at it this way, even if you are trying to be helpful, there are certain things you probably don't know about your diabetic friend. Like their blood sugar number at the time they eat, how much insulin they have taken, how much they've exercised that day, or even if they are fighting a cold. You also probably don't know their A1c levels for the past few years and what kind of day they are having.

Case in point, my husband and I went out to dinner not too long ago with a friend I had not seen in ages. At the time of our meal, I injected the normal amount of insulin. The problem was, I was so busy talking and catching up that I really didn't eat very much. I checked my blood sugar after dinner and sure enough it had dipped to 70. My husband went to get me a sugar soda, and when he did my friend said, "What, now you have to take more insulin because you ate too much?"

She, incidentally, was a runner and felt that anyone that had diabetes didn't take care of their health. When I told her that my blood sugar was actually low and I was trying to raise it (not lower it) she just shrugged like she didn't care.

Still, her disgusted tone reminded me why I didn't see her that often!

Make sure you aren't the friend that your diabetic pal avoids.

#7
Encourage Your Friend's Healthy Lifestyle

We've talked earlier about being a part of the "diabetic police." The opposite of that is being supportive of your friend's healthy outlook. Sometimes diabetics already have a healthy lifestyle when they get diabetes. Others change their way of life after diagnosis to take better care of themselves.

Regardless of where your friend is on the path to being healthy, encourage their progress. Celebrate their victories with a nice long walk after dinner.

Offer to work out with them when they go to the gym. If you have your diabetic friend over for dinner, make sure there is a nice variety of healthy foods.

If your friendship is centered around meals and "treats" (such as stopping for coffee or sugary snacks), change things up with something non-food related such as movies or sports. Suggest a spa or massage to relieve stress, rather than drinking or indulging in junk food.

Who knows, your friend's diagnosis may inspire you to get healthier, too!

#8
Be There for Your Friend

With any chronic disease, the greatest stress is simply the fact that no matter how well you take care of yourself, the disease is still there. Always. Some days it's better and some it's more of a struggle. But you never get a break.

Not a minute goes by where a diabetic doesn't think or act or feel something having to do with this disease that descended upon his or her body.

With all this happening, sometimes we just need someone to listen and be there for us.

Not all of us fall into a full-blown depression about having diabetes. But we do get down occasionally, and during those times it's nice to have someone that cares about us there to say, "I wish you didn't have to deal with this."

When we are down and want to share with you, give us your undivided attention and listen with all your heart. Just listen.

#9
Don't Talk About People Who Have Had Complications

When I tell someone I'm diabetic, one of two things happen. Either they immediately tell me about someone they know who has the disease, or they tell me about someone who lost a foot, or had a leg amputated, or went blind....

If you find that you have an urge to blurt out all the gory details of someone you know who has dealt with complications, let me tell you right now that we don't want to hear it. It's downright rude and besides that, it scares us.

Just because we're not walking around saying, "I'm worried one day that I could go blind" doesn't mean that it hasn't crossed our minds. The first thing you realize when you become diabetic is all the really nasty things that can happen to you.

And guess what? It's frightening. The thought of dealing with one of the numerous complications diabetics can suffer on top of the everyday maintenance really can become too much sometimes.

That's why, as our friend, we hope you will support us. We know you probably don't mean to scare us with bloody talk of kidney problems, nerve damage, or lost limbs. But you do. So simply keep those details to yourself and resist the urge to tell your friend every horror story you can. We'll be secretly glad you did.

#10
Make Sure You Have Plenty of Sugar-Free Beverages Around

When I first got diagnosed with diabetes, I was amazed at how many of my friends invited me over and never had anything but regular soda in their fridge. When I'd ask if they had diet, they'd simply say, "Oh I never drink that stuff!"

They weren't trying to be rude, of course, but when you invite over your diabetic friend it's a wonderful gesture to have some sugar-free soda or juices available. (So much better than offering them tap water!)

Even if your diabetic friend has a glass of wine or beer, always have some sugar-free drinks on hand since they probably won't want to drink alcohol all night. Trust me, they'll appreciate the gesture.

#11
Be Thankful For Your Own Good Health

The key word here is *thankful* (not arrogant.) As I've said, diabetes can strike the healthiest of people, so if you are one of the lucky ones blest with great health, be thankful.

How can that help your friend with diabetes? That's easy. When you admit how fortune you are to live without chronic disease, you are also acknowledging all those other people who aren't quite so lucky.

Besides that, there's nothing worse than seeing someone with perfectly good health not take care of themselves. So when you're thankful for the great body you've been given, it's more likely you will take care of it properly. And that, as your friend, makes us happy. We want to see you healthy, too.

#12
Don't Talk About How Diabetes Is "Almost Cured"

Granted, we've made huge strides in research and know more about diabetes than at any other time in history. That's exciting.

Moreover, we *are* getting close to a cure. That's even more exciting.

But it's not here yet.

I worked with someone who knew me when I was first diagnosed with diabetes. This was about twenty years ago. She saw me in the early stages when I was very sick and first adjusting to shots and insulin dosage. At the time I told her of my diagnosis she said, "Well you won't have it for long. They are close to a cure."

As twenty more years went on, she'd ask how I was doing and before I could answer would say, "Well diabetes is almost cured now." She'd say this even if we weren't talking about our health. It felt almost dismissive. It also made me wonder why she even asked how I was doing because she never waited for an answer.

And let me tell you, I'm not one to gripe about having diabetes. I've struggled at times. Like many diabetics, I also got other diseases like thyroid problems once I was diagnosed with diabetes. Every time I've been sick or had surgery or broke a bone I had diabetes to deal with in addition to the rest of my recovery.

Still, I don't complain. But one reason I wanted to write this book is because I'll bet there are a lot of people out there just like me who deal with diabetes and shrug off unhelpful and sometimes rude comments from people. And you know what? It doesn't have to be that way.

More importantly, the danger in talking too fast and loose about a cure is that it gives people the impression that we don't need funding or research for diabetes any longer. That is just not the case.

The words "close" to a cure can mean a lot of things. Just because a scientist says it's "close" doesn't mean all of us will be able to benefit from it. It could be years, decades, or longer. It could happen with a breakthrough overnight.

But even if they find a cure, it doesn't mean every diabetic will be able to live like "normal." It doesn't mean those folks with complications won't have them any longer.

Instead of talking about the cure, see what you can do to make it happen. Donate money. Volunteer. And in the meantime, support your pal with what they have to deal with now, and pray for a cure.

#13
Get Used to Seeing Test Supplies and Needles

If you are around your friend long enough, you are going to see him or her test their blood sugar or even give themselves insulin. When they do this, don't immediately start talking about how you hate needles or even how you "could never do that."

If you had diabetes you could. You would have to. Just like your friend.

No one relishes the thought of injecting themselves with a needle several times a day in order to live. But since your friend has to do it, support them.

Most diabetics will go into the bathroom when it comes to doing their shot, but every once in a while it isn't possible and they have to do it wherever they are. When this happens, don't make an issue of it. If the sight of needles makes you squeamish, simply turn your head. A shot only takes a few seconds to do.

#14
Be Cognizant of Dinner Times and Meal Planning

Part of a diabetics' job in learning how to live is timing. They have to time their insulin shots to coincide with their meal. Advancements in types of insulin have given diabetics more flexibility, but there will be times when your friend needs to eat now rather than later.

It's important, especially when inviting your diabetic friend along to dinner or when hosting a party, to let them know about what time the meal will be complete so a diabetic knows when to time their shots.

Before I started taking the short-acting insulin I'm on now, I used to take a kind that had to be in my system several minutes before the meal in order to work as it should. One my family members would invite my husband and I over for dinner, and tell us dinner will be ready at say, 6:00. I'd take my insulin as appropriate, only to find that at 6:00 she hadn't even started dinner and it would closer to 8:00 by the time we'd really sit down to eat.

The result was that I would have to drink juice for two hours and constantly monitor my blood sugar to keep it from dropping dangerously low. Then, when dinner would finally be ready, my insulin timing was off and my blood sugar would wind up high. All of that could have been avoided if she would have only been respectful of my medical needs.

To that end, there are also times when your diabetic friend will have to stop and rest or have a snack.   Every diabetic regime is different, depending on what the patient and doctor work out in terms of medication and meal planning. Talk to your friend to find out what kind of routine will suit their needs.

#15
Don't Say You "Wish You Had Diabetes So You Couldn't Eat Sugar"

As utterly ridiculous as this sounds, you'd be surprised how many times someone has said this to me. I'm not sure if there are folks who really believe that if they were diagnosed with diabetes they would say no to sugar easier, or if these people were trying to be supportive in a really twisted way.

Regardless of their intent, saying this is the equivalent of telling someone they are "lucky to have diabetes because it's easier to diet that way."

Diabetes doesn't help you say no to sugar. A good diabetes diet is a healthy, balanced diet. That's what everyone should aim for.

#16
Learn How to Test Blood Sugar and Give Shots

This is a big request for friends and family of diabetics, but I list this here because of my own experience. Until I met my husband, I was the only one giving me my shots. I developed certain "hardened" spots on my stomach because of the multiple shots I gave myself each day for twenty years.

When I met my husband, he volunteered to learn how to give me shots. The fact that he cared about me so much that he wanted to learn about my daily injections touched my heart. But more than that, it was like a weight lifted off of me.

Even though I still give myself the majority of my shots, knowing that someone else in my life is willing to do this for me is a tremendous blessing. More than that, it really helps when it comes to rotating injection sites.

Testing blood sugar for someone can also help if they are too sick to do it for themselves. Remember to always consult a diabetes professional to properly learn how to test blood sugar and do shots.

#17
Appreciate the Maintenance Required for Diabetes

It's rare when I sit down and tell someone everything I go through with diabetes. But the reality is, it's so much more than just "not eating sugar."

For example, while I have encountered many wonderful doctors and nurses, I have also had to deal with medical professionals who were extremely uneducated about the disease. Sometimes these people will recite "lower your blood sugar" by rote but won't have a clue about insulin shots or even current research.

I even had one physician's assistant tell me that the reason my blood sugar seemed to creep up in the morning was because I must be sneaking out of bed and eating sugar during the night. When I assured her this was not the case, she told me I must be lying. Anyone that knows anything about diabetes knows exactly why some diabetics have higher readings in the morning. All this person had to do was read a current issue of any one of the many diabetes magazines on the market to find that out.

As diabetics we have to be diligent about our health for many reasons. Dealing with misinformed medical professionals is just one of them. Another thing we deal with is insurance companies. There have been countless times I've tried to fill a prescription for insulin, only to have my pharmacy tell me the insurance company is "having a glitch" and won't fill it that day. This is insulin, mind you, something I need to survive each day.

The costs of diabetes can be just as difficult as managing the disease itself. Paying for insulin, needles, test strips, and blood glucose monitors is no easy task, especially when an insurance company doesn't cover all the costs to manage your disease.

Diabetics deal with a lot of things as a result of having this disease. It can be frustrating to the point of distraction. We can spend hours on the phone trying to correct a problem. All of this takes a toll on our health.

But with friends to support us, it lets us know that we have someone in our corner.

#18
Attend a Diabetic Support Group With Your Friend

Getting diabetes can be a scary thing to deal with at first. But more than that, diabetics need to take in a lot of information just to be able to live.

When we are first diagnosed, diabetics are strongly encouraged to bring their family to "diabetic classes." The classes are usually held on weekends and last a couple of hours. In these classes, diabetics and their families learn things like how and when to take medications, how to deal with stress in a healthy way, and how to eat right.

Most times a diabetic's family is very supportive of their disease, and will willingly attend the "diabetic class" with them. Some diabetics, like yours truly, have parents and family that can't be bothered to attend the classes with them. More than that, they'll be dismissive if the diabetic even tries to explain all the things they have to do in order to live.

Getting a diagnosis like diabetes without emotional support can be devastating. If your diabetic friend lacks emotional support during these early days, offer to attend their classes and support group with them. I can't tell you how much they will appreciate your kindness. It may make all the difference in how they approach the disease going forward.

#19
Get Involved

It's one thing to get information about diabetes, it's another to really become involved in the fight for a cure.

I can tell you for a fact that I personally appreciate every person who volunteers or raises money or gets involved with walks. I am humbled and grateful for any effort people may put in on behalf of diabetes. I know other diabetics are as well.

There are so many times you feel alone in the effort to manage your diabetes, that hearing that there are people out there helping to bring awareness makes each and every one of us feel a bit less alone in our struggle.

And is it really a struggle?

It can be, yes. Even the most in-control diabetics have days where they are sick of blood sugars and testing and needles. They're sick of complications and working so hard to do what everyone else seems to be able to do without thinking. For one day, they'd like to be able to go out the door and take a walk without thinking about having glucose tablets or testing materials on hand.

On those days, we look to all of you who help in the fight for a cure and silently say, "Thank you."

#20
Call Out Anyone Who
is Misinformed

The best way to stop the spread of ridiculous beliefs is through education. You don't need to teach a class in order to make this happen. If you hear someone make an assumption about diabetes that is not true, correct them. Make sure people understand that the things they say and do have an impact, so they should at least get the proper knowledge before talking about diabetes.

Diabetics deal with many things, including healthcare costs, daily injections, and a body that sometimes doesn't cooperate. They don't need to deal with people who talk about things they don't understand as well.

#21
Become a Diabetes Advocate

You'd be surprised at how easy it is to be a diabetes advocate. The American Diabetes Association (ADA), especially, has made it very simple to become involved by contacting your senators and congressmen. The ADA provides links to the elected officials in your area, how to get in touch with them, and what to say.

They also provide information on which issues are currently being discussed in Washington, what they mean for diabetics, and what you can do to help.   For more information, visit the ADA's website: http://www.diabetes.org/.

About the Author

Cherie Burbach is a poet, mixed media artist, and freelance writer specializing in lifestyle and relationships. She's written for About.com, NBC/Universal, Match.com, Christianity Today, and more. Visit her website for more info, cherieburbach.com.

ISBN 978-0-9789747-7-0

www.ingramcontent.com/pod-product-compliance
Lightning Source LLC
Chambersburg PA
CBHW051038030426
42336CB00015B/2940